Undifferentiated Connective Tissue Disease

A Beginner's 3-Step Plan to Managing UCTD Through Diet, with Sample Recipes and a Meal Plan

mf

copyright © 2022 Patrick Marshwell

All rights reserved No part of this book may be reproduced, or stored in a retrieval system, or transmitted in any form or by any means, electronic, mechanical, photocopying, recording, or otherwise, without express written permission of the publisher.

Disclaimer

By reading this disclaimer, you are accepting the terms of the disclaimer in full. If you disagree with this disclaimer, please do not read the guide.

All of the content within this guide is provided for informational and educational purposes only, and should not be accepted as independent medical or other professional advice. The author is not a doctor, physician, nurse, mental health provider, or registered nutritionist/dietician. Therefore, using and reading this guide does not establish any form of a physician-patient relationship.

Always consult with a physician or another qualified health provider with any issues or questions you might have regarding any sort of medical condition. Do not ever disregard any qualified professional medical advice or delay seeking that advice because of anything you have read in this guide. The information in this guide is not intended to be any sort of medical advice and should not be used in lieu of any medical advice by a licensed and qualified medical professional.

The information in this guide has been compiled from a variety of known sources. However, the author cannot attest to or guarantee the accuracy of each source and thus should not be held liable for any errors or omissions.

You acknowledge that the publisher of this guide will not be held liable for any loss or damage of any kind incurred as a result of this guide or the reliance on any information provided within this guide. You acknowledge and agree that you assume all risk and responsibility for any action you undertake in response to the information in this guide.

Using this guide does not guarantee any particular result (e.g., weight loss or a cure). By reading this guide, you acknowledge that there are no guarantees to any specific outcome or results you can expect.

All product names, diet plans, or names used in this guide are for identification purposes only and are the property of their respective owners. The use of these names does not imply endorsement. All other trademarks cited herein are the property of their respective owners.

Where applicable, this guide is not intended to be a substitute for the original work of this diet plan and is, at most, a supplement to the original work for this diet plan and never a direct substitute. This guide is a personal expression of the facts of that diet plan.

Where applicable, persons shown in the cover images are stock photography models and the publisher has obtained the rights to use the images through license agreements with third-party stock image companies.

Table of Contents

Introduction
What Is UCTD?
    UCTD Symptoms
    UCTD Causes
    Diagnosis of Undifferentiated Connective Tissue Disease (UCTD)
    Treating UCTD
    Lifestyle Changes for UCTD

The UCTD Diet
    Principles of a UCTD Diet
    Benefits of a UCTD Diet
    Disadvantages of a UCTD Diet

3-Step Plan to Manage the UCTD Diet
    Step 1: Engage the Help of a Doctor or Dietician
    Step 2: Meal Planning
    Step 3: Mindful Eating
    Foods to Eat
    Foods to Avoid
    Other methods and approaches to managing UCTD

Sample Recipes
    Roasted Chicken Thighs
    Roasted Chicken
    Ginger Chicken Stir Fry
    Salmon and Asparagus
    Seafood Stew
    Baked Salmon
    Apple and Onion Soup
    Asian-Style Vegetable Soup
    Meaty Cauliflower Soup

    Keto Pesto Chicken
    Cauliflower Pizza
    Baked Tuna and Asparagus
    Apricot-Glazed Salmon
    Barley Oat Pancakes
    Blackberry Cobbler
    Quinoa and Vegetable Stir-Fry
    Salmon and Avocado Salad
    Chickpea and Spinach Curry
    Sweet Potato and Black Bean Tacos
    Blueberry Chia Pudding
    Roasted broccoli and Salmon

Sample Meal Plan
Conclusion
FAQs
References and Helpful Links

Introduction

Undifferentiated Connective Tissue Disease (UCTD) is a term used to categorize a group of conditions that exhibit some, but not all, characteristics of more commonly recognized connective tissue diseases. Currently, there isn't comprehensive data on the number of Americans diagnosed with UCTD. However, based on small case studies by researchers, it's estimated that about 72% of UCTD patients are White, and approximately 78% are female.

This disease involves the immune system erroneously attacking the body's tissues. Although UCTD shares symptoms with various connective tissue diseases, these symptoms don't align specifically with any one disease. While UCTD has sometimes been labeled as Mixed Connective Tissue Disease (MCTD), some experts argue that they are distinct clinical entities.

Nutrition plays a crucial role in supporting and enhancing the immune system, and for individuals with UCTD, it is a vital component in managing the disease. Alongside nutritional strategies, other natural methods are often employed to improve the quality of life for those with UCTD. The key to maintaining a healthy and prolonged life is working closely with a healthcare provider to identify what works best for your body and finding effective ways to alleviate and prevent symptoms.

In this quick-start beginner's guide, you will discover the following:

- All about UCTD
- What causes UCTD
- Diagnosing and treating UCTD
- The UCTD diet
- Ways to manage UCTD and stick to the diet
- A 3-step plan

Keep reading to learn more about UCTD and how to manage it through nutrition and other natural methods.

What Is UCTD?

UCTD, or undifferentiated connective tissue disease, is a term used to describe a group of autoimmune diseases that share some common symptoms but have not yet been fully classified. This term in the early days of medical discovery identified people who had symptoms of early-stage connective disease but didn't meet the standard criteria for diagnosis of any particular connective tissue disease.

Some connective tissue diseases with known symptoms and criteria for diagnosis include systemic lupus erythematosus, rheumatoid arthritis, systemic sclerosis, Sjogren's syndrome, etc. UCTD can affect any organ or system in the body, and there is currently no cure.

Autoimmune diseases are caused by the body's immune system attacking healthy cells and tissues. There are over 80 different autoimmune diseases, and many of them are still relatively unknown to the medical community. Some of the patients with UCTD present with symptoms that are seen in lupus while others have symptoms seen in other types of connective tissue diseases.

Some even present with a combination of symptoms from two or more types of connective tissue diseases. Undifferentiated connective tissue disease is different from mixed connective tissue disease. Some patients may remain undifferentiated for life or experience a remission of symptoms while others may progress to having only the symptoms of differentiated connective tissue disease.

Autoimmune diseases can affect any part of the body, from the muscles and joints to the digestive system and brain. They can be extremely debilitating and often require lifelong treatment. There is no one-size-fits-all approach to managing autoimmune diseases, but a combination of medication, lifestyle changes, and dietary modifications is usually required. There is still much to learn about autoimmune diseases, and researchers are working hard to find new treatments and cures.

UCTD Symptoms

Undifferentiated Connective Tissue Disease (UCTD) is a term used to describe autoimmune diseases that have features of connective tissue diseases but do not meet the full criteria for any specific one. Symptoms can vary widely and may include:

- *General Symptoms*: These can include persistent fatigue that doesn't go away with rest, recurring fevers, and unintentional weight loss. It's important to monitor these symptoms as they can be indicative of underlying conditions.

- *Joint and Muscle Pain*: Often presenting with arthritis-like symptoms such as stiffness, swelling, and pain in the joints. Myalgia, or muscle pain, can also occur, leading to general discomfort and reduced mobility.
- *Skin Symptoms*: This may involve various types of rashes, most notably a butterfly-shaped rash that spans across the cheeks and nose. Additionally, there may be heightened sensitivity to sunlight (photosensitivity), causing skin irritation or rashes upon exposure. Raynaud's phenomenon is another common issue, where fingers or toes change color (white, blue, then red) when exposed to cold or stress.
- *Nail Changes*: Observations may include red or inflamed cuticles, pitting, ridges, or other abnormalities in the nails, which can be signs of systemic issues.
- *Oral Ulcers*: These are typically painless sores that appear inside the mouth. They might go unnoticed but are noteworthy symptoms to report to a healthcare provider.
- *Lung Issues*: Difficulty breathing, coughing, and chest pain may occur if lung tissue is affected. Inflammation of the lung lining (pleuritis) and scarring of lung tissue (pulmonary fibrosis) are also possible.

- ***Heart Problems***: This can manifest as pericarditis, an inflammation of the pericardium (the double-walled sac containing the heart). Symptoms might include sharp chest pain, fever, and a feeling of overall malaise.

It's important to recognize and document these symptoms, as they can provide critical clues for diagnosing and managing various health conditions. If you experience any of these symptoms, consulting with a healthcare provider is advised.

These symptoms can fluctuate and may evolve over time, sometimes leading to a more definitive diagnosis of a specific connective tissue disease. If you or someone you know is experiencing these symptoms, it is important to consult a healthcare professional for evaluation and management.

UCTD Causes

The exact causes of Undifferentiated Connective Tissue Disease (UCTD) are not well understood, but several factors are believed to contribute to its development:

- ***Genetic Factors***: A family history of autoimmune diseases can increase the risk of developing UCTD. Certain genetic markers and predispositions may play a role.
- ***Immune System Dysfunction***: Autoimmune responses, where the body's immune system mistakenly attacks its

own tissues, are central to UCTD. The specific mechanisms triggering this response are still under investigation.

- ***Environmental Triggers***: External factors such as infections (viral or bacterial), stress, exposure to certain chemicals, and ultraviolet (UV) light exposure can act as triggers in genetically predisposed individuals.
- ***Hormonal Influences***: Hormones may influence the development and progression of UCTD, especially since the disease is more common in women, suggesting a potential link with hormonal changes.
- ***Infections***: Some infections might trigger an abnormal immune response that could lead to autoimmune conditions like UCTD.
- ***Tobacco Use***: Smoking has been associated with an increased risk of developing various autoimmune diseases, including those related to connective tissue.

Understanding and identifying these factors can help in managing and potentially preventing UCTD, but ongoing research is necessary to fully elucidate the underlying causes. If you suspect you have UCTD, a healthcare professional can provide a more comprehensive evaluation and guidance.

Diagnosis of Undifferentiated Connective Tissue Disease (UCTD)

Diagnosing Undifferentiated Connective Tissue Disease (UCTD) involves a combination of clinical evaluation, laboratory tests, and sometimes imaging studies. Here are the key steps typically involved in the diagnosis:

1. **Clinical Evaluation**: A comprehensive medical history and physical examination are conducted to assess symptoms and signs associated with connective tissue diseases. This includes evaluating joint pain, skin rashes, Raynaud's phenomenon, and other relevant symptoms.
2. **Laboratory Tests**:
    - *Antinuclear Antibody (ANA) Test*: A positive ANA test is common in UCTD and other autoimmune conditions. It indicates the presence of autoantibodies directed against the cell nucleus.
    - *Specific Autoantibodies*: Tests for specific autoantibodies such as anti-dsDNA, anti-Ro/SSA, anti-La/SSB, anti-Smith, and anti-RNP may be performed to rule out other connective tissue diseases.
    - *Inflammatory Markers*: Elevated levels of markers like ESR (erythrocyte sedimentation

rate) and CRP (C-reactive protein) can indicate inflammation.
3. **Exclusion of Other Conditions**: UCTD is diagnosed when the patient exhibits signs and symptoms of a connective tissue disease but does not meet the full criteria for a specific condition such as systemic lupus erythematosus (SLE), rheumatoid arthritis, or scleroderma. Physicians carefully rule out these diseases through clinical criteria and specific antibody profiles.
4. **Monitoring Over Time**: Since UCTD can evolve into a more specific connective tissue disease, patients are often monitored over time. Follow-up visits and repeated testing are important to observe any changes in symptoms or laboratory results.
5. **Imaging Studies**: In some cases, imaging studies such as X-rays, ultrasound, or MRI may be used to assess joint or organ involvement.
6. **Referral to Specialists**: Consultation with a rheumatologist, a specialist in autoimmune and connective tissue diseases, is often necessary for a definitive diagnosis and appropriate management.

The diagnosis of UCTD requires a nuanced approach, considering both clinical presentation and laboratory findings to ensure accurate identification and effective management of the condition.

Treating UCTD

There is no one-size-fits-all approach to treating UCTD, but a combination of medication, lifestyle changes, and dietary modifications are usually required.

Medication for UCTD may include NSAIDs (nonsteroidal anti-inflammatory drugs) or corticosteroids to help reduce inflammation.

Lifestyle Changes for UCTD

Lifestyle changes can play a significant role in managing Undifferentiated Connective Tissue Disease (UCTD). Here are some key lifestyle modifications that can help improve symptoms and overall well-being:

1. **Diet and Nutrition**
   - *Balanced Diet*: Focus on a diet rich in fruits, vegetables, whole grains, lean proteins, and healthy fats. This helps support overall health and reduce inflammation.
   - *Limit Trigger Foods*: Keep a food diary and note any foods that worsen symptoms. Avoid or limit these trigger foods to manage UCTD symptoms.
   - *Hydration*: Drink plenty of water to stay hydrated and support bodily functions.

- ***Limit Processed Foods***: Reduce intake of processed foods, sugary snacks, and beverages, which can contribute to inflammation.

2. **Regular Exercise**
   - ***Low-Impact Activities***: Engage in low-impact exercises like walking, swimming, or cycling to maintain joint mobility and overall fitness without putting excessive stress on the joints.
   - ***Strength Training***: Incorporate gentle strength training exercises to build muscle support around the joints.
   - ***Flexibility Exercises***: Practice stretching and flexibility exercises, such as yoga or tai chi, to improve range of motion and reduce stiffness.

3. **Stress Management**
   - ***Mindfulness and Meditation***: Techniques like mindfulness meditation, deep-breathing exercises, and progressive muscle relaxation can help manage stress and reduce its impact on symptoms.
   - ***Counseling and Support Groups***: Participating in therapy or support groups can provide emotional support and coping strategies from others who understand the challenges of living with UCTD.

4. **Skin Protection**
   - ***Sun Protection***: Use sunscreen with high SPF, wear protective clothing, and seek shade to protect against photosensitivity and skin rashes triggered by UV exposure.
   - ***Moisturizing***: Regularly moisturize your skin to prevent dryness and irritation.
5. **Healthy Sleep Habits**
   - ***Regular Sleep Schedule***: Aim for a consistent sleep schedule by going to bed and waking up at the same time each day.
   - ***Sleep Environment***: Create a comfortable and quiet sleep environment to promote restful sleep.
   - ***Sleep Hygiene***: Avoid caffeine and electronic devices before bedtime to improve sleep quality.
6. **Avoiding Triggers**
   - ***Smoking Cessation***: If you smoke, seek help to quit, as smoking can exacerbate symptoms and increase the risk of complications.
   - ***Environmental Factors***: Identify and avoid environmental triggers, such as exposure to cold temperatures (which can worsen Raynaud's phenomenon) or certain chemicals.

7. **Regular Medical Check-Ups**
   - *Follow-Up Visits*: Keep regular appointments with your healthcare provider to monitor your condition and adjust treatment as needed.
   - *Vaccinations*: Stay up-to-date with recommended vaccinations to prevent infections that could trigger flare-ups.
8. **Energy Conservation**
   - *Pacing*: Learn to pace your activities and take breaks when needed to avoid overexertion.
   - *Prioritizing Tasks*: Focus on important tasks and delegate or postpone less critical activities to conserve energy.

These lifestyle changes, when combined with medical treatment, can help manage symptoms, reduce flare-ups, and enhance the quality of life for individuals with UCTD. Always consult with your healthcare provider before making significant changes to your lifestyle or treatment plan.

The UCTD Diet

Diet is a major natural tool for managing UCTD symptoms. Eating a balanced diet and maintaining proper nutrition supports immune function and helps relieve some symptoms. Many people have reported fewer crises with UCTD. Besides general health benefits, a good diet can prevent other chronic diseases affecting UCTD sufferers.

There are no specific diet rules for UCTD, but those with autoimmune disorders are generally advised to avoid certain foods and incorporate more of others. The focus is on a simple, sustainable diet.

They should also avoid substances that affect the immune system or trigger inflammation. A good diet helps sustain energy, nourish organs, maintain muscle mass, prevent unhealthy weight gain, and promote overall well-being. Some evidence suggests a gluten-free diet may improve UCTD symptoms. Gluten is a protein found in wheat, barley, and rye. If you have celiac disease or gluten sensitivity, avoid foods containing gluten.

Principles of a UCTD Diet

The principles of a UCTD (Undifferentiated Connective Tissue Disease) diet are centered around reducing inflammation, supporting the immune system, and promoting overall well-being. Here are the key principles to keep in mind:

1. *Anti-inflammatory Foods*: Incorporate foods known for their anti-inflammatory benefits, including fruits, vegetables, nuts, seeds, and oily fish. These foods can help reduce inflammation, which is a common issue in connective tissue diseases.
2. *Omega-3 Fatty Acids*: Omega-3 fatty acids are essential for overall health and can help reduce inflammation in the body. Sources of omega-3s include oily fish such as salmon, chia seeds, flaxseeds, and walnuts.
3. *Whole Grains*: Choose whole grains like quinoa, brown rice, oats, and whole wheat over refined grains. Whole grains provide essential nutrients and fiber, which support digestive health and stabilize blood sugar levels.
4. *Lean Proteins*: Opt for lean proteins such as chicken, turkey, beans, legumes, and plant-based protein sources. These proteins are important for muscle repair and overall health without contributing to inflammation.

5. ***Fresh Fruits and Vegetables***: Aim for a variety of colorful fruits and vegetables, which are rich in vitamins, minerals, and antioxidants. These nutrients help combat oxidative stress and inflammation.
6. ***Healthy Fats***: Include healthy fats from sources like olive oil, avocados, and nuts. These fats support cell health and reduce inflammation.
7. ***Hydration***: Stay well-hydrated by drinking plenty of water throughout the day. Proper hydration supports overall bodily functions and can help manage symptoms.
8. ***Limit Processed Foods***: Minimize the intake of processed foods, which often contain unhealthy fats, sugars, and additives that can exacerbate inflammation and other symptoms.
9. ***Avoid Trigger Foods***: Identify and avoid foods that may trigger symptoms. Common triggers can include gluten, dairy, and certain additives, but these can vary between individuals.
10. ***Balanced Meals***: Strive for balanced meals that combine lean proteins, healthy fats, and complex carbohydrates to maintain stable energy levels and support overall health.
11. ***Mindful Eating***: Practice mindful eating by paying attention to how foods affect your body. Keep a food diary to track symptoms and identify potential triggers.

12. ***Consistency***: Maintain a consistent eating schedule to help regulate metabolism and prevent unnecessary stress on the body.

By following these principles, you can create a diet that not only helps manage UCTD symptoms but also promotes overall health and well-being. Always consider consulting with a healthcare professional or a nutritionist to tailor these guidelines to your specific needs.

Benefits of a UCTD Diet

Adopting a UCTD (Undifferentiated Connective Tissue Disease) diet can offer numerous benefits that go beyond symptom management. Here are some of the key advantages:

1. ***Reduced Inflammation***: A primary benefit of a UCTD diet is the reduction of inflammation in the body. Incorporating anti-inflammatory foods can help manage and alleviate inflammation, which is a core issue in connective tissue diseases.
2. ***Improved Immune Function***: Nutrient-dense foods rich in vitamins, minerals, and antioxidants can strengthen your immune system. This support is crucial for individuals with UCTD, as it can help the body better regulate immune responses and reduce flare-ups.
3. ***Enhanced Energy Levels***: Consuming balanced meals that include lean proteins, whole grains, and healthy

fats can stabilize blood sugar levels and provide sustained energy throughout the day. This can help combat fatigue, which is a common symptom among those with UCTD

4. ***Better Digestion***: A diet high in fiber from fruits, vegetables, and whole grains can promote digestive health. Proper digestion is essential for nutrient absorption and can help prevent gastrointestinal issues often linked with UCTD.

5. ***Weight Management***: Maintaining a healthy weight is easier with a diet focused on whole, unprocessed foods. Proper weight management can relieve stress on joints and tissues, which is particularly beneficial for UCTD patients.

6. ***Joint and Muscle Health***: Including anti-inflammatory foods in your diet and consuming fatty fish and leafy greens can alleviate joint pain and stiffness associated with UCTD. Additionally, nutrients like calcium and vitamin D from dairy products or fortified plant-based alternatives can support bone health.

7. ***Improved Mental Health***: A nutritious diet can stabilize mood and reduce the risk of depression and anxiety, which are sometimes experienced by individuals dealing with chronic illnesses like UCTD.

8. ***Cardiovascular Health***: Healthy fats, whole grains, and a diet low in processed foods contribute to heart

health. This is important for UCTD patients as they may be at an increased risk for cardiovascular issues.
9. *Skin Health*: A diet rich in antioxidants and healthy fats can improve skin health, which can be significant since UCTD can sometimes affect the skin.
10. *Long-Term Health Benefits*: Adhering to a UCTD diet can have long-term health benefits, including reduced risk of chronic diseases such as diabetes, cardiovascular disease, and certain cancers.
11. *Personalized Nutrition*: By focusing on foods that your body responds well to and avoiding known triggers, you can create a nutrition plan tailored to your specific needs. This personalized approach ensures that your diet is not only effective but also enjoyable.
12. *Empowerment and Control*: Taking charge of your diet empowers you to play an active role in managing your condition. Knowing that you can make choices that positively impact your health can provide a sense of control and optimism.

Overall, a UCTD diet is more than just a way to manage symptoms; it's a holistic approach to improving overall quality of life. By fueling your body with the right foods, you can enhance your physical health, emotional well-being, and long-term vitality.

Disadvantages of a UCTD Diet

While the UCTD (Undifferentiated Connective Tissue Disease) diet offers numerous benefits, it's also important to recognize that there may be some challenges or disadvantages associated with it. However, it's crucial to keep in mind that the benefits often outweigh these drawbacks.

1. ***Time-Consuming Meal Preparation***: Adopting a UCTD diet often involves preparing meals from scratch using fresh, whole ingredients. This can be time-consuming, especially for those with busy schedules or limited energy. However, investing time in meal preparation ensures that you consume nutrient-dense foods that support your health and well-being.
2. ***Higher Grocery Costs***: Whole, fresh, and organic foods can sometimes be more expensive than processed alternatives. While this might strain your budget, the long-term investment in your health can reduce medical expenses and improve your quality of life, making the cost worthwhile.
3. ***Social and Convenience Challenges***: Sticking to a specific diet can be challenging in social situations where food options may not align with your dietary needs. It may require extra planning and communication with hosts or restaurants. Despite this, the benefits of adhering to your diet, such as reduced

symptoms and improved well-being, can make these efforts worthwhile.

4. ***Limited Food Choices***: A UCTD diet may involve avoiding certain foods that trigger symptoms, which can sometimes feel restrictive. This might limit your food choices and require creativity in meal planning. However, focusing on the wide variety of delicious and nutritious foods you can enjoy can make your diet feel less restrictive and more enjoyable.

5. ***Learning Curve***: Transitioning to a UCTD diet involves learning new recipes, understanding nutritional information, and possibly changing long-standing eating habits. This learning curve can be daunting initially, but over time, these new habits can become second nature, leading to sustainable and beneficial lifestyle changes.

6. ***Need for Meal Planning***: Effective meal planning is essential to ensure you're getting a balanced intake of nutrients. This requires effort and organization. However, having a plan helps prevent impulsive eating choices that might not align with your dietary goals, ultimately supporting better health.

7. ***Adjusting to New Flavors and Textures***: Shifting to a diet high in fruits, vegetables, and whole grains might mean getting used to new flavors and textures. Some people may find this adjustment challenging at first.

Nevertheless, discovering new foods and enjoying their health benefits can be a rewarding experience.

8. ***Potential for Nutrient Deficiencies***: If not carefully planned, any restrictive diet has the potential to result in nutrient deficiencies. Working with a nutritionist can help ensure that you're meeting all your nutritional needs, thereby turning this potential disadvantage into an opportunity for personalized and informed dietary choices.

Despite these challenges, the overall benefits of a UCTD diet—such as reduced inflammation, improved immune function, enhanced energy levels, better digestion, and long-term health improvements—far outweigh these disadvantages. By addressing these challenges head-on with thoughtful planning and professional guidance, you can effectively manage your UCTD symptoms while enjoying a healthier, more vibrant life.

3-Step Plan to Manage the UCTD Diet

There are a few natural methods or approaches that are recommended by different researchers or physicians in the management of UCTD symptoms. Dieting is one of the most popular natural approaches to UCTD management and for good reason. There have been reports of a reduction in symptoms, flare-ups, and improvement in quality of life amongst several people living with UCTD.

Using dieting as a plan for managing UCTD will involve working with a health expert particularly a doctor or a dietician to create meal plans that are appropriate and sustainable for the individual. It is important to always remember that the same plan doesn't work for everyone. Understanding what works for your body system is the first step and you cannot achieve that without a good plan.

A 3-step plan to manage UCTD through diet

Step 1: Engage the Help of a Doctor or Dietician

This is an important step that lays a strong foundation for your journey towards better health and nutrition. With the sheer volume of dietary recommendations available online and the various pieces of advice from well-meaning friends, family, and even influencers, it can be overwhelming to discern what is truly beneficial for your unique needs. While these sources may offer general guidance, they often lack the personalized touch that is crucial for making informed decisions about your diet.

To ensure that you are making the right choices and not depriving your body of essential nutrients, the first and most critical step is to engage the help of a professional. A doctor or a registered dietician possesses the expertise and experience necessary to navigate the complexities of nutrition. They can provide you with tailored advice that considers your medical history, lifestyle, and specific health goals.

Working with a healthcare professional ensures that any dietary changes you make are safe and effective. They can help you identify any nutritional deficiencies you may have and recommend foods or supplements to address them. Additionally, they can assist you in creating a balanced meal plan that promotes overall well-being without compromising on taste or variety.

The process of understanding what works for you and determining which foods are best to incorporate into your daily diet should be undertaken with their guidance. This collaborative approach allows for adjustments and fine-tuning based on your body's responses, ensuring that your dietary habits support long-term health and vitality. By prioritizing this step, you set yourself up for success, armed with the knowledge and confidence that comes from professional support.

Step 2: Meal Planning

Meal planning is a crucial component in maintaining a healthy, varied, and nutrient-dense diet, especially for those dealing with Undifferentiated Connective Tissue Disease (UCTD). The goal is to ensure you are not stuck in a cycle of repetitive, dull, and nutritionally insufficient meals. Effective meal planning involves thoughtfully selecting and organizing your daily menu in advance, which helps streamline shopping, simplify food preparation, and promote a sustainable long-term eating strategy.

Benefits of Meal Planning

By planning your meals ahead of time, you can enjoy several benefits:

1. *Reduced Stress*

Knowing what you'll eat each day eliminates the last-minute scramble to figure out meal options and reduces daily decision fatigue. This allows you to focus your energy on other important tasks and responsibilities, such as work projects, family time, or personal hobbies. Additionally, planning meals ahead can help you ensure a balanced diet, avoid unhealthy fast food choices, and save money by reducing food waste.

2. *Improved Nutrition*

Planning allows you to incorporate a variety of nutrient-dense foods into your diet, ensuring a balanced intake of essential vitamins and minerals. This can lead to better overall health and improved energy levels, contributing to a more vibrant lifestyle.

3. *Cost Efficiency*

Meal planning helps you avoid unnecessary purchases and reduces food waste, making your grocery shopping more efficient and budget-friendly. By sticking to a list, you limit impulse buys and can take advantage of bulk purchases and sales, saving money over time.

4. *Health Management*

For patients with Undifferentiated Connective Tissue Disease (UCTD), incorporating anti-inflammatory foods into meal plans can help manage symptoms and improve overall well-being. Consistently eating a balanced diet with these specific nutrients can reduce flare-ups and support a healthier immune system.

5. *Creative Recipe Exploration*

Before diving into meal planning, it's beneficial to explore a variety of recipes that align with a UCTD diet. Look for dishes that incorporate the foods allowed on your list in diverse and enjoyable ways. This not only keeps your meals interesting but also ensures you're getting the nutrients your body needs.

6. *Anti-Inflammatory Foods*

Include foods recognized for their anti-inflammatory benefits, such as fatty fish like salmon and mackerel, leafy greens such as spinach and kale, nuts like walnuts and almonds, seeds such as flaxseeds and chia seeds, and fruits like strawberries, blueberries, and raspberries. These foods can help reduce inflammation, improve overall health, and manage UCTD symptoms effectively.

7. *Nutrient-Dense Choices*

Focus on foods rich in vitamins, minerals, and antioxidants to support your immune system and overall well-being. Whole grains (such as quinoa, brown rice, and oats), lean proteins (like chicken, turkey, and tofu), and a variety of fresh fruits and vegetables (including those high in vitamins C and E) should be staples in your diet. These nutrient-dense options provide the essential nutrients your body needs to function optimally and combat inflammation.

Weekly and Daily Meal Planning

Plan your meals on a weekly basis, breaking them down into daily menus. This approach allows you to maintain variety while ensuring you meet your nutritional needs.

1. *Keep It Simple*

   Complexity can lead to burnout. Choose simple yet delicious recipes that are easy to prepare and fit within your financial constraints. Opt for one-pot meals or dishes that require minimal ingredients, and don't shy away from utilizing kitchen gadgets like slow cookers or instant pots to save time and effort.

2. *Sustainable Practices*

   Creating a sustainable meal plan is key. This involves using staple ingredients that you can buy in bulk and store easily, such as frozen vegetables, fresh frozen fruits, pureed tomatoes, and pre-cooked proteins like shrimp and chicken. Additionally, focus on seasonal produce and locally sourced items to not only support local farmers but also ensure freshness and reduce your carbon footprint. Plan your meals in advance to minimize food waste and make the most out of your groceries.

Organizing Your Meal Plan

To make meal planning even more efficient, consider creating a menu book and recipe collection. This resource can serve as your go-to guide for meal ideas and shopping lists, ensuring you always have the ingredients you need on hand.

1. *Stock Your Pantry*

   Keep essential items stocked, so you're never caught off guard. Staples like whole grains, legumes, and frozen produce are versatile and can be used in numerous recipes. Additionally, having a variety of spices and condiments can enhance the flavor of your dishes, making it easier to create delicious meals even on short notice.

2. *Flexibility*

   Allow for flexibility in your meal plan to accommodate changes in your schedule or unexpected cravings. Having a backup plan can help you stay on track without feeling restricted. For instance, keep a list of quick and easy recipes that you enjoy and can prepare with minimal ingredients. This way, you can adapt your meal plan to suit your mood or any last-minute changes in your day.

By investing time in meal planning, you set yourself up for success in managing UCTD through a balanced diet. Not only will you enjoy a variety of delicious, nutritious meals, but you'll also support your overall health and well-being.

Step 3: Mindful Eating

Mindful eating is an essential practice for anyone, especially for those managing Undifferentiated Connective Tissue Disease (UCTD). By being intentional about your eating habits, you can significantly improve your overall health and manage your symptoms more effectively. Here's how you can integrate mindful eating into your daily routine:

Building and Maintaining Intentional Eating Habits

Planning your meals lays the groundwork for mindful eating. It helps you become more aware of what you consume and enables you to make better food choices.

1. *Food Diary*

    Keeping a food diary can be incredibly beneficial. Documenting what you eat throughout the day allows you to monitor your meal patterns, track your nutrient intake, and identify any foods that may trigger symptoms. By noting down the time, portion sizes, and even your mood while eating, you gain valuable insights into your eating habits and can make more informed dietary decisions.

2. *Avoid Mindless Shopping*

Shop with a list and stick to it. Impulse buys often lead to unhealthy food choices that can derail your diet plan. Plan your meals in advance, create a detailed shopping list based on these meals, and avoid grocery shopping when you're hungry to prevent temptation.

3. *Consistent Mealtimes*

Schedule your meal times and try to adhere to them as closely as possible. Skipping meals or changing your eating schedule frequently to eat out or grab a quick snack can lead to poor food choices and unbalanced nutrition. Consistent mealtimes help regulate your metabolism and ensure that your body gets the nutrients it needs at regular intervals.

Making Thoughtful Choices

Each meal is an opportunity to nourish your body. Consider the importance of what you eat at every mealtime, and make thoughtful decisions that align with your dietary goals.

1. *Avoid Unplanned Eat-Outs*

Spontaneous meals out can often lead to consuming unhealthy foods and derailing your dietary goals. To combat this, try to avoid unplanned restaurant visits or fast-food runs by preparing your meals in advance and sticking to your meal schedule. Meal prepping on weekends or the night before can ensure you have healthy options readily available, reducing the temptation to eat out.

2. *Stay on Plan*

When dining out for a lunch or dinner meeting, keep your diet plan in mind. Many restaurants offer healthier options or accommodations for specific dietary needs—don't hesitate to ask for modifications to fit your UCTD diet. For instance, you could request dressing on the side, grilled instead of fried options, or even inquire about low-sodium or gluten-free dishes. Planning ahead by checking the menu online before you arrive can also help you make better choices.

Benefits of Homemade Meals

For people living with UCTD, homemade meals are usually the best option. Preparing your food gives you complete control over what goes into your meals, ensuring they meet the recommendations of your dietician and do not contain any ingredients that may trigger flare-ups.

1. *Custom-Tailored to Your Needs*

Homemade meals allow you to cook according to your taste preferences while adhering to your diet plan. You can use fresh, whole ingredients that support your health without worrying about hidden additives or allergens. Additionally, you have the flexibility to experiment with different recipes, ensuring that your meals are both nutritious and enjoyable.

2. *Easier Tracking*

When you prepare your meals, it's easier to track what you eat and monitor portion sizes. This level of control is crucial for maintaining a balanced diet and managing UCTD effectively. By keeping a detailed food diary, you can better understand your nutritional intake, identify potential triggers, and make informed adjustments to your diet as needed.

By committing to mindful eating, you can enhance the effectiveness of your meal-planning efforts. Being intentional about your food choices, keeping a structured eating schedule, and prioritizing homemade meals will help you stay on track with your UCTD diet and promote better health outcomes.

To improve the healthiness of your meals; the method of preparation is also very important. Here are some helpful tips:

1. Make use of more fresh products when possible. Avoid canned foods or products.

2. Make use of healthy oils like olive oil, canola oil, flax oil, etc.
3. Choose an air fryer over frying foods in oil or fat
4. Incorporate lots of vegetables in your meals
5. Stay away from seasonings heavy on salt. Go for salt-free seasoning blends and fresh herbs for seasoning your dishes.

Foods to Eat

A diet that supports managing Undifferentiated Connective Tissue Disease (UCTD) should focus on anti-inflammatory and nutrient-dense foods. Here are some recommended foods to include:

1. ***Fruits and Vegetables***: Rich in antioxidants, vitamins, and minerals. Examples include berries, leafy greens, broccoli, carrots, and citrus fruits.
2. ***Omega-3 Fatty Acids***: Found in fatty fish like salmon, tuna, and sardines. These healthy fats have anti-inflammatory benefits that can help reduce UCTD symptoms.
3. ***Whole Grains***: Such as brown rice, quinoa, oats, and whole wheat. They provide fiber and essential nutrients.
4. ***Lean Proteins***: Includes poultry, tofu, beans, lentils, and fish. These are important for muscle maintenance and repair.

5. ***Nuts and Seeds***: Almonds, walnuts, chia seeds, and flaxseeds offer healthy fats, protein, and fiber.
6. ***Healthy Fats***: Avocados, olive oil, and nuts are great sources of monounsaturated and polyunsaturated fats.
7. ***Legumes***: Beans, lentils, and chickpeas are high in fiber, protein, and essential nutrients.
8. ***Herbs and Spices***: Turmeric, ginger, garlic, and cinnamon have anti-inflammatory benefits.
9. ***Fermented Foods***: Such as yogurt, kefir, sauerkraut, and kimchi. These can promote gut health.
10. ***Hydration***: Plenty of water and herbal teas to stay hydrated and support overall health.

Incorporating these foods into your diet may help manage symptoms and improve overall health. Always consider consulting with a healthcare provider or nutritionist to tailor a diet that meets your specific needs and conditions.

Foods to Avoid

When managing Undifferentiated Connective Tissue Disease (UCTD) through diet, it is generally recommended to avoid certain foods that may exacerbate inflammation or interfere with the immune system. Here are some foods to consider avoiding:

1. ***Processed Foods***: These often contain additives, preservatives, and unhealthy fats that can increase inflammation.

2. **Refined Sugars**: Foods high in refined sugars can lead to inflammation and metabolic issues. This includes candy, pastries, and sugary beverages.
3. **Trans Fats**: Found in many fried foods, baked goods, and margarine, trans fats can contribute to inflammation.
4. **Red and Processed Meats**: High consumption of red meats and processed meats like sausages and bacon has been linked to increased inflammation.
5. **Gluten**: Some individuals with UCTD may find that gluten exacerbates their symptoms, so it might be helpful to try a gluten-free diet.
6. **Dairy Products**: For some people, dairy can cause inflammation and digestive issues. This varies from person to person.
7. **Nightshade Vegetables**: These include tomatoes, eggplants, peppers, and potatoes. Some people with autoimmune conditions report worsened symptoms with these foods.
8. **Alcohol**: Excessive alcohol consumption can increase inflammation and negatively affect the immune system.
9. **High Sodium Foods**: Too much salt can aggravate inflammation and contribute to hypertension.
10. **Artificial Sweeteners**: Certain artificial sweeteners may upset the gut microbiome and potentially increase inflammation.

It's important to note that dietary triggers can vary significantly between individuals. It may be beneficial to work with a healthcare provider or a nutritionist to tailor a diet plan that best suits your specific needs and conditions.

Other methods and approaches to managing UCTD

These methods are usually used in combination with dieting and other medical therapies and lifestyle adjustments to manage UCTD symptoms and improve the quality of life.

1. **Stress Management**

    To effectively manage stress, it's important to make lifestyle changes that incorporate relaxation activities and to take breaks from work when it becomes overwhelming. Engaging in mind-soothing activities like listening to music, practicing yoga, dancing, and similar pursuits can help mitigate the harmful effects of stress on your body. Remember, it's perfectly okay to take vacations and rest.

2. **Exercise and Physical Activity**

    Exercise is a cornerstone of a healthy lifestyle, and this is especially true for individuals living with UCTD. Regularly engaging in simple exercises a few times a week helps to build muscle strength and reduce the risk of several chronic diseases. Prioritizing physical activity is essential for maintaining overall well-being.

Several organizations offer support systems for helping people living with UCTD and with the help of your doctor, you can get in touch with them to get the benefits that their activities offer. Joining support groups also provides you with a safe space to cope with the mental and physical strains of the condition.

Sample Recipes

We know that planning meals can be challenging, especially when you have UCTD. Here are a few easy and delicious recipes loaded with nutrients perfect for individuals living with UCTD:

Roasted Chicken Thighs

Ingredients:

- 12 garlic cloves, unpeeled
- 1 tbsp. avocado oil
- 1 pinch of Himalayan pink salt
- 4 chicken thighs with skin
- 1 tsp. Primal Palate super gyro seasoning

Instructions:

1. Pour avocado oil over a medium-sized oven-safe pot.
2. Add the garlic cloves. Sauté over medium heat for 2 to 3 minutes or until the skins begin to brown.
3. Place the chicken in a large skillet over medium-high heat. Sear for about 2 to 3 minutes for each side, starting with the skin side.
4. Combine the chicken with the garlic. Season generously with salt and Primal Palate Super Gyro seasoning.
5. Place the chicken in an oven preheated to 350°F.
6. Bake for one hour while covered.
7. Serve and enjoy.

Roasted Chicken

Ingredients:

- 1 whole organic chicken
- 2 sprigs of organic rosemary
- 2 garlic cloves
- 1 tbsp. herbes de Provence
- 1 tbsp. coarse sea salt

Instructions:

1. Preheat your oven to 425°F.
2. Rinse the chicken and pat dry with paper towels.
3. Loosen the skin over each breast by gently pushing your fingers between the skin and meat, being careful not to tear the skin.
4. Slice one garlic clove into thin slices and place them under the skin on top of each breast, along with a sprig of rosemary.
5. Crush the remaining garlic clove and rub it all over the chicken's surface.
6. Sprinkle herbes de Provence and coarse sea salt evenly over the chicken's surface.
7. Place the chicken in a roasting pan and roast for 30 minutes.
8. After 30 minutes, reduce the oven temperature to 375°F and continue roasting for an additional 45

minutes, or until the internal temperature of the thickest part of the thigh reaches 165°F.
9. Let the chicken rest for at least 10 minutes before carving and serving.

Enjoy your delicious roast chicken with your favorite sides!

Ginger Chicken Stir Fry

Ingredients:

Stir-fry mix:

- 1 lb. cooked chicken, dark or light meat
- 4 cups cremini mushrooms, sliced
- 4 cups purple cabbage, sliced
- 2 cups carrots
- 1/2 cup green onions, cut slanted
- 3 cups cauliflower florets
- 1 handful of enoki mushrooms
- 2 tbsp. avocado oil
- 1 package of rice noodles, cook according to instructions

Stir-fry sauce:

- 4 cloves minced garlic
- 1/4 cup honey
- 1/4 tsp. grated ginger
- 1/4 cup rice wine vinegar
- 1 tsp. favorite hot sauce
- 1 cup chicken stock
- 1 tbsp. avocado oil

Instructions:

1. Slice the cremini mushrooms, purple cabbage, and carrots. Cut the green onions at a slant. Break the

cauliflower into florets. Have the cooked chicken ready, either dark or light meat, depending on your preference.
2. Prepare the rice noodles according to the package instructions. Once cooked, drain and set aside.
3. In a bowl, combine the minced garlic, honey, grated ginger, rice wine vinegar, hot sauce, chicken stock, and 1 tablespoon of avocado oil. Mix well until all ingredients are fully incorporated.
4. In a large skillet or wok, heat 2 tablespoons of avocado oil over medium-high heat.
5. Add the sliced cremini mushrooms, purple cabbage, carrots, green onions, cauliflower florets, and enoki mushrooms to the skillet. Stir-fry for about 5-7 minutes, or until the vegetables are tender but still crispy.
6. Add the cooked chicken to the skillet with the vegetables. Stir-fry for another 2-3 minutes to ensure the chicken is heated through.
7. Pour the prepared stir-fry sauce over the chicken and vegetable mixture. Stir well to coat all ingredients evenly. Let it cook for an additional 3-5 minutes, allowing the sauce to thicken slightly.

8. Add the cooked rice noodles to the skillet. Toss everything together until the noodles are well coated with the sauce and mixed with the vegetables and chicken.
9. Serve the ginger chicken stir-fry hot, straight from the skillet. Enjoy this nutritious and flavorful dish!

Salmon and Asparagus

Ingredients:

- 2 salmon filets
- 14-oz. young potatoes
- 8 asparagus spears, trimmed and halved
- 2 handfuls cherry tomatoes
- 1 handful basil leaves
- 2 tbsp. extra-virgin olive oil
- 1 tbsp. balsamic vinegar

Instructions:

1. Heat oven to 428°F.
2. Arrange potatoes into a baking dish.
3. Drizzle potatoes with extra-virgin olive oil.
4. Roast potatoes until they have turned golden brown.
5. Place asparagus into the baking dish together with the potatoes.
6. Roast in the oven for 15 minutes.
7. Arrange cherry tomatoes and salmon among the vegetables.
8. Drizzle with balsamic vinegar and the remaining olive oil.
9. Roast until the salmon is cooked.
10. Throw in basil leaves before transferring everything to a serving dish.
11. Serve while hot.

Seafood Stew

Ingredients:

- 2 tsp. extra-virgin olive oil
- 1 cut bulb fennel
- 2 stalks celery, chopped
- 2 cups white wine
- 1 tbsp. chopped thyme
- 1 cup chopped shallots
- 6 ounces shrimp
- 6 ounces of sea scallops
- 1/4 tsp. salt
- 1 cup chopped parsley
- 6 oz. Arctic char
- 2-1/2 cups of water

Instructions:

1. Heat a frying pan on the lowest setting. Add a small amount of oil.
2. Cook the celery, shallots, and fennel for approximately 6 minutes.
3. Pour the wine, water, and thyme into the frying pan.
4. Wait for 10 minutes and allow it to cook.
5. Once much of the water has evaporated, add in the remaining ingredients, and wait for 2 minutes before removing it from the stove.
6. Serve and enjoy immediately.

Baked Salmon

Ingredients:

- 2 salmon fillets
- 6 cups of fresh spinach
- 2 tsp. coconut oil
- 1/4 tsp. garlic powder
- 1/4 tsp. turmeric
- 3 large cloves of garlic
- lemon juice
- salt
- pepper

Instructions:

1. Preheat the oven to 400°F.
2. Line a baking dish with parchment paper.
3. Marinate salmon fillets in lemon juice, coconut oil, garlic powder, turmeric, salt, and pepper.
4. Let it sit for a few minutes. This may also be done the night before to help the juices and flavor get into the salmon.
5. Once the oven is ready, bake the salmon for 15 minutes.

6. Cook some of the garlic in a pan with coconut oil.
7. Add spinach and cook until ready. Season with salt and pepper to taste.
8. Take salmon out of the oven and put spinach beside it.
9. Serve and enjoy.

Apple and Onion Soup

Ingredients:

- 3 organic apples, diced
- 2 medium yellow onions, sliced
- 6 cups vegetable broth
- 1 small leek, chopped
- 1 tbsp. avocado oil
- 1/2 tbsp. fresh rosemary, chopped
- 1/2 tbsp. fresh thyme

Instructions:

1. In a large pot, heat avocado oil over medium heat.
2. Add sliced onions and cook until they are slightly caramelized.
3. Add in diced apples, chopped leeks, rosemary, and thyme. Cook for 5 minutes.
4. Pour in vegetable broth and bring to a boil.
5. Reduce heat to low and let it simmer for 20 minutes.
6. Once the soup has thickened, remove it from the heat and let it cool.
7. Using an immersion blender or regular blender, blend soup until smooth.
8. Serve hot with a sprinkle of fresh herbs on top for garnish.

Asian-Style Vegetable Soup

Ingredients:

- 1/3 large head of cabbage, shredded
- 1 medium or large head of bok choy, stem and leaves separated
- 9 artichoke hearts, drained
- 2 cups beef or venison, boiled and cubed
- 6 cups beef broth, preferably homemade
- 4 cups leafy green vegetables, chopped
- 1/3 lb. fresh or frozen broccoli, chopped
- 2 large organic carrots, sliced or diced
- 5 oz. water chestnuts, drained and diced or sliced
- 2 medium onions, sliced or diced
- 4 cloves garlic, minced
- 1/2-in. to 3-in. fresh ginger root, grated
- 2-4 tbsp. fat
- 1-1/2 tsp. rock salt or kosher salt
- ground black pepper, to taste
- 1 cup cauliflower, chopped

Instructions:

1. Melt your preferred fat using medium heat in a pot.
2. Sauté the onions for at least 5 minutes.
3. Stir in bok choy stems.
4. Continue stirring until onions and bok choy are translucent.

5. Add the garlic, carrots, cabbage, and ginger.
6. Stir around for 1 to 2 minutes.
7. Add the bok choy leaves and any other leafy green vegetables
8. Stir and cover for about a minute.
9. Pour in the beef broth.
10. Increase the heat to high.
11. Add the salt, pepper, artichokes, and meat.
12. Cover the pot with its lid.
13. Add broccoli, cauliflower, and water chestnuts.
14. When the broth comes to a boil, reduce the heat to medium-low.
15. Cook for 5 to 15 minutes.
16. Serve hot with a side of soy sauce or grated cheese.

Meaty Cauliflower Soup

Ingredients:

- 1 cup cauliflower, chopped
- 1/8 tsp. pepper
- 1/8 tsp. ground mustard
- 1 chicken stock
- 2-1/2 cups hot water
- fresh parsley, chopped

Instructions:

1. Heat a saucepan. Pour in water and condensed chicken broth.
2. Add cauliflower, mustard, and pepper.
3. Stir from time to time.
4. Adjust heat to high. Let it boil.
5. Reduce the heat. Allow it to simmer while covered.
6. Stir from time to time until the potatoes are soft.
7. Add ham and add in half and half.
8. Cook for 5 more minutes, uncovered. Do not boil.
9. Turn off the heat as soon as the soup starts to simmer.
10. Top with parsley upon serving.

Keto Pesto Chicken

Ingredients:

- 1-1/2 lbs chicken thighs breasts, boneless and cut into bite-sized pieces
- pepper
- salt
- 2 tbsp. butter or coconut oil
- 5 tbsp. red or green pesto
- 1-1/4 cups heavy whipping cream
- 5 oz. feta cheese, diced
- 3 oz. pitted olives
- 1 garlic clove, finely chopped

Salad:

- 5 oz. leafy greens
- 4 tbsp. olive oil
- sea salt
- ground black pepper

Instructions:

1. Preheat the oven to 400°F.
2. Season the chicken with salt and pepper.
3. Add butter or oil to a large skillet. Fry the chicken pieces on medium-high heat until golden brown.
4. In a bowl, combine heavy cream and pesto. Mix well.

5. Put the fried chicken meat in a baking dish. Add in olives, garlic, and feta cheese.
6. Pour the pesto or cream mixture.
7. Bake in the oven for 20-30 minutes.
8. Toss all the salad ingredients upon serving.
9. Serve and enjoy.

Cauliflower Pizza

Ingredients:

- cauliflower
- 1/4 cup of tomato pasta sauce
- 1/4 cup of pesto sauce (no sugar)
- 100 grams of thinly sliced mozzarella
- 250 grams of cut tomatoes
- 2-3 medium-sized eggs
- basil leaves

Instructions:

1. Preheat oven to 425°F.
2. Cut the cauliflower into small pieces and place them in a food processor until it forms a rice-like texture.
3. Cook the cauliflower rice for about 5 minutes on medium heat, stirring occasionally. Let cool afterward.
4. Once cooled, mix in the eggs with the cauliflower "dough".
5. Spread parchment paper on top of a baking sheet and evenly spread out the mixture onto it forming a circular shape.
6. Bake for 15-20 minutes or until it turns slightly golden brown.
7. Once done, let it cool down before spreading tomato sauce over the cauliflower crust.

8. Spread the pesto sauce on top and add sliced mozzarella and tomatoes as toppings.
9. Put back in the oven for an additional 10 minutes or until the cheese is melted and bubbly.
10. Sprinkle fresh basil leaves on top before serving.
11. Enjoy your healthy and delicious cauliflower pizza!

Baked Tuna and Asparagus

Ingredients:

- 2 5-oz. tuna fillets
- 14 oz. young potatoes
- 8 asparagus spears, trimmed and halved
- 2 handfuls of cherry tomatoes
- 1 handful fresh basil leaves
- 2 tbsp. extra-virgin olive oil
- 1 tbsp. balsamic vinegar

Instructions:

1. Heat oven to 428°F.
2. Arrange potatoes in a baking dish. Drizzle with a tablespoon of extra-virgin olive oil.
3. Roast potatoes for 20 minutes, or until golden brown.
4. Place the asparagus into the baking dish together with the potatoes. Roast in the oven for another 15 minutes.
5. Arrange the cherry tomatoes and tuna among the vegetables. Drizzle with balsamic vinegar and the remaining olive oil.
6. Roast for 10 to 15 minutes, or until tuna is cooked.
7. Throw in a handful of basil leaves before transferring everything to a serving dish. Serve while hot.

Apricot-Glazed Salmon

Ingredients:

- 1-1/3 pounds wild salmon filets
- 1/4 tsp. of crushed black pepper*
- 1 tbsp. virgin olive oil
- 1/2 cup of sodium-free vegetable broth
- 1 tbsp. Dijon mustard
- 1/3 cup of 100% apricot fruit spread
- 1 tsp. minced garlic

Instructions:

1. Preheat the grill over medium heat.
2. Pat salmon dry with a paper towel and cut it into four slices.
3. Season the skinless side with black pepper.
4. Wrap each piece with aluminum foil, with the skin side down. Fold the foil around the salmon securely to prevent oil from leaking.
5. In a bowl, combine the remaining ingredients.
6. Pour the mixture over the salmon slices.
7. Grill salmon for ten minutes.
8. Once cooked, allow the grilled filet to cool down before unwrapping.
9. Plate nicely and garnish with your favorite herbs before serving.

*black pepper may be substituted with white pepper.

Barley Oat Pancakes

Ingredients:

- 1 cup barley flour
- 1 cup oat flour
- 1 tbsp. baking powder, sodium-free
- 1 tsp. salt
- 1-1/2 cup nonfat milk
- 2 pcs. large eggs
- 2 tbsp. canola oil
- 2 tbsp. honey
- 2 tsp. vanilla extract
- honey or maple syrup, for serving
- your choice of fresh fruit

Instructions:

1. In a large mixing bowl, whisk together the oat flour, barley flour, salt, and baking powder.
2. In a separate mixing bowl, whisk together the eggs, oil, non-fat milk, vanilla extract, and honey.
3. Transfer the wet ingredients to the large mixing bowl. Whisk them together to combine. Do not overmix the batter.
4. Place a large non-stick pan over low-medium heat.
5. Put about 3 tablespoons of batter into the pan. Wait for bubbles to appear on the top side of the pancake and for the bottom to turn golden brown.

6. Flip the pancake to cook the other side.
7. Repeat until all the batter is cooked.
8. Top each pancake with your choice of fresh fruit.
9. Drizzle honey or maple syrup over the fruit.
10. Serve the pancakes immediately.

Blackberry Cobbler

Ingredients:

- 2 tbsp. organic coconut oil, with an additional amount for greasing
- 1/4 cup arrowroot flour
- 12 oz. blackberries
- 1/4 cup raw honey
- 3 tbsp. water
- 1/4 tsp. salt
- 1-1/4 tsp. lemon juice
- 3/4 tsp. baking soda
- 1/4 cup coconut flour

Instructions:

1. Preheat the oven to 300°F.
2. Use coconut oil to grease an 8×8 baking dish.
3. Place blackberries at the bottom of the pan, ensuring that they are placed evenly.
4. Place the remaining ingredients in a food processor. Pulse at medium speed until thoroughly combined and then spread over blackberries.
5. Bake for 35 to 40 minutes or until the top turns golden brown.
6. Serve and enjoy.

Quinoa and Vegetable Stir-Fry

Ingredients:

- 1 cup quinoa
- 2 cups water
- 1 tablespoon olive oil
- 1 onion, chopped
- 2 cloves garlic, minced
- 1 bell pepper, chopped
- 1 zucchini, sliced
- 1 cup broccoli florets
- 1 carrot, sliced
- 2 tablespoons soy sauce or tamari (for gluten-free)
- Juice of 1 lemon
- Salt and pepper to taste

Instructions:

1. Rinse quinoa under cold water. Combine quinoa and water in a pot and bring to a boil. Reduce heat, cover, and simmer for 15 minutes until quinoa is tender.
2. In a large pan, heat olive oil over medium heat. Add onion and garlic, and sauté until translucent.
3. Add bell pepper, zucchini, broccoli, and carrot. Stir-fry for about 5-7 minutes until vegetables are tender but still crisp.

4. Add cooked quinoa to the vegetables and mix well.
5. Stir in soy sauce and lemon juice. Season with salt and pepper to taste.
6. Serve warm.

Salmon and Avocado Salad

Ingredients:

- 2 salmon fillets
- 1 tablespoon olive oil
- Salt and pepper to taste
- 4 cups mixed greens (spinach, arugula, kale)
- 1 avocado, sliced
- 1 cucumber, sliced
- 1/4 cup red onion, thinly sliced
- 2 tablespoons pumpkin seeds
- Juice of 1 lemon
- 2 tablespoons extra-virgin olive oil
- 1 teaspoon Dijon mustard

Instructions:

1. Season salmon fillets with salt and pepper. Heat olive oil in a pan over medium-high heat. Cook salmon for 4-5 minutes on each side until fully cooked. Let it cool slightly and then flake into pieces.
2. In a large bowl, combine mixed greens, avocado, cucumber, red onion, and pumpkin seeds.

3. In a small bowl, whisk together lemon juice, extra-virgin olive oil, and Dijon mustard.
4. Drizzle dressing over the salad and toss gently to combine.
5. Top the salad with flaked salmon and serve immediately.

Chickpea and Spinach Curry

Ingredients:

- 1 tablespoon coconut oil
- 1 onion, chopped
- 3 cloves garlic, minced
- 1 tablespoon ginger, grated
- 1 can (15 oz) chickpeas, drained and rinsed
- 1 can (14 oz) diced tomatoes
- 1 can (14 oz) coconut milk
- 4 cups fresh spinach
- 2 teaspoons curry powder
- 1 teaspoon ground cumin
- 1 teaspoon ground turmeric
- Salt and pepper to taste
- Fresh cilantro, chopped (optional)

Instructions:

1. In a large pan, heat coconut oil over medium heat. Add onion, garlic, and ginger, and sauté until onion is translucent.
2. Add chickpeas, diced tomatoes, and coconut milk. Stir well to combine.
3. Add curry powder, cumin, turmeric, salt, and pepper. Simmer for 10-15 minutes until the sauce thickens.
4. Stir in fresh spinach and cook until wilted.
5. Serve hot, garnished with chopped cilantro if desired.

Sweet Potato and Black Bean Tacos

Ingredients:

- 2 large sweet potatoes, peeled and cubed
- 2 tablespoons olive oil
- 1 teaspoon paprika
- 1 teaspoon ground cumin
- Salt and pepper to taste
- 1 can (15 oz) black beans, drained and rinsed
- 1 avocado, diced
- 1/4 cup red onion, chopped
- Corn tortillas
- Fresh lime wedges
- Fresh cilantro, chopped (optional)

Instructions:

1. Preheat oven to 400°F (200°C). Toss sweet potato cubes with olive oil, paprika, cumin, salt, and pepper. Spread on a baking sheet and roast for 25-30 minutes until tender.
2. Warm corn tortillas in a dry skillet or oven.
3. In a bowl, combine roasted sweet potatoes, black beans, avocado, and red onion.
4. Fill each tortilla with the sweet potato mixture.
5. Serve with fresh lime wedges and garnish with chopped cilantro if desired.

Blueberry Chia Pudding

Ingredients:

- 1/4 cup chia seeds
- 1 cup almond milk (or any preferred milk)
- 1 tablespoon maple syrup
- 1 teaspoon vanilla extract
- 1 cup fresh blueberries
- 2 tablespoons crushed almonds (optional)

Instructions:

1. In a jar or container, mix chia seeds, almond milk, maple syrup, and vanilla extract. Stir well to combine.
2. Let the mixture sit for at least 30 minutes to allow the chia seeds to absorb the liquid and thicken into a pudding-like consistency.
3. In a blender, blend fresh blueberries until smooth.
4. Layer the chia pudding and blueberry puree in serving glasses or jars.
5. Top with crushed almonds if desired.
6. Refrigerate for at least an hour before serving to allow flavors to meld together.
7. Serve chilled as a healthy breakfast or snack option.

Roasted broccoli and Salmon

Ingredients:

- 1 head broccoli, cut into florets
- 2 salmon fillets
- 2 tablespoons olive oil
- Salt and pepper to taste
- Lemon wedges for serving (optional)

Instructions

1. Preheat oven to 400°F (200°C). Line a baking sheet with parchment paper.
2. In a bowl, toss broccoli florets with olive oil, salt, and pepper.
3. Place the broccoli on one side of the baking sheet and place the salmon fillets on the other side.
4. Drizzle olive oil over the salmon and season with salt and pepper.
5. Roast in the oven for 15-20 minutes, until salmon is cooked through and broccoli is tender.
6. Serve with lemon wedges if desired for added flavor.

Sample Meal Plan

There are several recommendations online and from health professionals on how to develop a great diet plan to manage UCTD. Every person has different needs so the same plan will not work for everyone. The diet plan has to work for you, reduce your saturated fat intake, reduce your intake of processed foods, and increase the intake of healthy foods. The meal plan you work with should reduce stress and maintain a healthy balanced diet sustainable for a long time.

Here is a sample meal plan featuring healthy dishes that work for a UCTD diet. The recipes are provided in Chapter 4.

Breakfast: *Meaty Cauliflower Soup* - light enough to serve as a perfect breakfast choice and loaded with enough calories and nutrients to provide a nourishing replacement for several other regular breakfast options.

Lunch: *Ginger Chicken Stir-fry* - a delicious and very nutritious sauce that can be served with rice noodles to make a beautiful lunch option.

Snack: Healthy salad made from leafy greens, olive oil, sea salt, and a little ground black pepper. Instead of processed sugars, candies, cakes, cookies, and so on, a healthy snack made up of veggies is advised for a UCTD diet.

Dinner: *Roasted broccoli and Salmon* - this is a light and nutritious dinner featuring fish that is rich in omega-3 fatty acids and veggies that are rich in nutrients.

Dessert: *Apple and onion soup* - if you must have something delicious as a dessert, try to keep it as healthy as possible and free from processed sugars and flour. Soup is a healthy choice that aids digestion and reduces gut inflammation. It is rich in nutrients that boost the immune system.

Several healthy UCTD meal recipes can fit into your daily meal plan. Switching up the unhealthy snack and dessert choices and staying away from fast food or junk is a very good start towards a healthier diet.

Conclusion

Thank you for taking the time to read our comprehensive guide on Undifferentiated Connective Tissue Disease (UCTD) and the UCTD diet. Your dedication to understanding this complex condition is commendable, and you should be proud of the knowledge you have gained. By equipping yourself with information, you are taking a significant step towards better managing your health or supporting someone who is navigating life with UCTD.

Living with UCTD can be challenging, but remember that knowledge is power. Understanding the symptoms, potential triggers, and treatment options allows you to make informed decisions that can enhance your quality of life. This journey is about more than just managing symptoms; it's about thriving despite them. As you implement the dietary recommendations discussed in this guide, you're not only aiming to alleviate symptoms but also promoting overall well-being.

Your diet plays a crucial role in managing UCTD. By focusing on nutrient-dense foods, you can support your immune system, reduce inflammation, and improve your energy levels. It's amazing how much of an impact small changes, like incorporating more fruits, vegetables, and whole grains, can have on your overall health. Avoiding processed foods and those high in sugar and trans fats can further help mitigate inflammation and other symptoms associated with UCTD.

Listening to your body is key. Pay attention to how different foods make you feel and adjust your diet accordingly. What works for one person may not work for another, and that's okay. The goal is to find a balance that suits your unique needs. Consult with healthcare professionals such as nutritionists or dietitians who can provide personalized advice tailored to your condition.

Beyond diet, consider integrating other lifestyle changes into your routine. Regular physical activity, adequate sleep, and stress management techniques like meditation or yoga can greatly support your overall health. Exercise, in particular, can help maintain joint flexibility and muscle strength, which is especially beneficial for individuals with connective tissue diseases.

It is essential to keep an open line of communication with your healthcare provider. Regular check-ups and being proactive about any new or worsening symptoms can significantly impact your treatment plan's effectiveness. Don't hesitate to ask questions or express concerns; your healthcare team is there to support you.

You're now equipped with valuable insights and practical strategies for managing UCTD. Remember, managing a chronic condition is a marathon, not a sprint. Patience and consistency are your allies. Celebrate your progress, no matter how small, and give yourself grace on days when things don't go as planned.

Your commitment to understanding UCTD and making positive changes in your life is truly inspiring. Continue to educate yourself, stay connected with support groups or communities, and most importantly, believe in your ability to live a fulfilling life despite the challenges.

Congratulations again on completing this guide. Your proactive approach to your health is commendable, and we hope the information provided empowers you to navigate your journey with confidence and resilience. Here's to your health, happiness, and continued success on your path to wellness.

FAQs

What is Undifferentiated Connective Tissue Disease (UCTD)?

UCTD is a type of autoimmune disorder where the immune system attacks the body's tissues, but it does not meet the full criteria for a specific connective tissue disease like lupus or rheumatoid arthritis. Symptoms can vary widely and may include joint pain, skin rashes, and fatigue.

Can diet help manage symptoms of UCTD?

While diet alone cannot cure UCTD, eating an anti-inflammatory and nutrient-rich diet can help manage symptoms, reduce inflammation, and support overall health.

What foods should I avoid if I have UCTD?

It is recommended to avoid processed foods, refined sugars, trans fats, red and processed meats, gluten, dairy products, nightshade vegetables, alcohol, high sodium foods, and artificial sweeteners as these can exacerbate inflammation.

What foods should I include in my diet to help manage UCTD?

Aim to incorporate foods that are rich in antioxidants, omega-3 fatty acids, and anti-inflammatory compounds. This encompasses fruits and vegetables (particularly leafy greens), fatty fish such as salmon or tuna, nuts and seeds, whole grains, legumes, and healthy fats like olive oil.

How can omega-3 fatty acids help with UCTD?

Omega-3 fatty acids, present in fatty fish, chia seeds, flaxseeds, and walnuts, are recognized for their anti-inflammatory benefits, which can help alleviate inflammation and manage symptoms related to UCTD.

Are there any specific dietary plans or guidelines for people with UCTD?

There isn't a one-size-fits-all dietary plan for UCTD. However, following a balanced diet that emphasizes anti-inflammatory foods, such as the Mediterranean diet, can be beneficial. It's best to work with a healthcare provider or nutritionist to create a personalized plan.

How important is hydration in managing UCTD?

Staying well-hydrated is crucial for overall health and can help manage UCTD symptoms. Drinking plenty of water and herbal teas supports bodily functions and helps maintain joint health.

References and Helpful Links

Connect, A. (2021, May 3). Mixed connective tissue Disease diet. Autoimmune Connect. https://drbonnie360.com/2018/11/09/food-spotlight-on-mixed-connective-tissue-disease/

Home—Genetic and rare diseases information center. (n.d.). Retrieved November 26, 2022, from https://rarediseases.info.nih.gov/.

Undifferentiated Connective Tissue Disease – In-Depth | HSS. (n.d.). Hospital for Special Surgery. https://www.hss.edu/conditions_undifferentiated-connective-tissue-disease-overview.asp

Tracy, L., PhD. (2024, February 16). Undifferentiated connective tissue disease. Rheumatology Advisor. https://www.rheumatologyadvisor.com/ddi/undifferentiated-connective-tissue-disease/

Cd-N, A. C. R. (2022, August 5). What to eat when you have mixed connective tissue disease. Verywell Health. https://www.verywellhealth.com/what-to-eat-when-you-have-mixed-connective-tissue-disease-5097156

Undifferentiated Connective Tissue Disease (UCTD): treatment. (n.d.). National Jewish Health. https://www.nationaljewish.org/conditions/uctd-undifferentiated-connective-tissue-disease/treatment#:~:text=Some%20medications%20that%20can%20be, clinical%20monitoring%20to%20ensure%20safety.

Johns Hopkins Lupus Center. (2019, March 27). Lifestyle and additional information : Johns Hopkins Lupus Center. https://www.hopkinslupus.org/lupus-info/lifestyle-additional-information/

Printed in Great Britain
by Amazon